Complete Guide to Intermittent Fasting

The Eating Pattern Making Weight Loss Possible While Eating the Foods You Want for Women and Men, Highly Effective Fasting Tips to Stay Slim Permanently

Christine Moore

© Copyright 2019 - All rights reserved.

The content contained within this book may not be reproduced, duplicated or transmitted without direct written permission from the author or the publisher.

Under no circumstances will any blame or legal responsibility be held against the publisher, or author, for any damages, reparation, or monetary loss due to the information contained within this book. Either directly or indirectly.

Legal Notice:
This book is copyright protected. This book is only for personal use. You cannot amend, distribute, sell, use, quote or paraphrase any part, or the content within this book, without the consent of the author or publisher.

Disclaimer Notice:
Please note the information contained within this document is for educational and entertainment purposes only. All effort has been executed to present accurate, up to date, and reliable, complete information. No warranties of any kind are declared or implied. Readers acknowledge that the author is not engaging in the rendering of legal, financial, medical or professional advice. The content within this book has been derived from various sources. Please consult a licensed professional before attempting any techniques outlined in this book.

By reading this document, the reader agrees that under no circumstances is the author responsible for any losses, direct or indirect, which are incurred as a result of the use of information contained within this document, including, but not limited to, — errors, omissions, or inaccuracies.

Contents

Introduction _____ 1

Chapter 1:
What is Intermittent Fasting? _____ 2

Chapter 2:
The Benefits of an Intermittent Fast _____ 12

Chapter 3:
Common Side Effects of Intermittent Fasting _____ 19

Chapter 4:
Choices for Intermittent Fasting _____ 23

Chapter 5:
Starving Yourself Vs Intermittent Fasting _____ 33

Chapter 6:
What Foods Should I Eat on An Intermittent Fast? _____ 38

Chapter 7:
The Safe Way to End Your Fast _____ 47

Chapter 8:
The Safe Way to Eat During Your Eating Window _____ 54

Chapter 9:
How to Prepare for Intermittent Fasting _____ 61

Chapter 10:
How to Get Back on Track if You Fall Off the Fast _____ 67

Chapter 11:
Exercising While Intermittent Fasting _____ 71

Chapter 12:
Tips to Stay Motivated and Success _____ 77

Chapter 13:
Common Questions _____ 84

Conclusion _____ 89

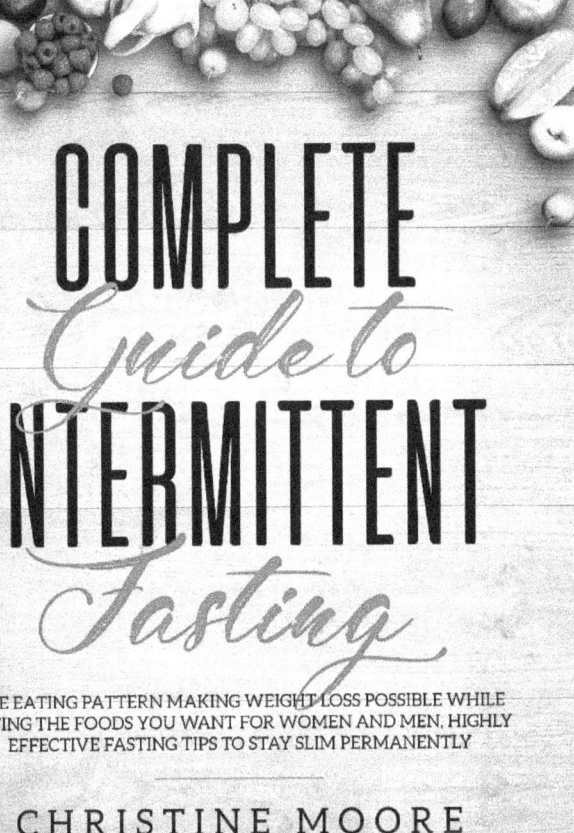

Introduction

The following chapters will discuss the important topics you need to know before getting started on an intermittent fast. Intermittent fasting is an important eating plan that can help you burn fat, limit your calories, and improve a whole host of different health issues. This guidebook will be your trusty tool to fully understand an intermittent fast and how to get started.

In this guidebook, we will look at the different aspects of an intermittent fast. We will look at what this fasting is, how it works better than other forms of dieting, some of the health benefits, what foods you should eat on the diet, how to figure out your daily calories, and more. When you finish this guidebook, you will be ready to get started with intermittent fasting on your own.

When you are ready to lose weight without having to religiously count calories, and you want to improve many different aspects about your health, check out this guidebook to help you learn more about an intermittent fast.

Chapter 1:
What is Intermittent Fasting?

Intermittent fasting is a way of eating that can help to improve your life and your health. While traditional calorie restriction can be hard on a person and can result in overeating and binging, intermittent fasting helps you to avoid the hunger pains and still lose weight.

The traditional American diet asks us to eat three meals a day, along with snacks. We are basically allowing ourselves to eat all day long. We have breakfast right when we wake up in the morning and often finish out the day with a little snack before bed.

This is seen as normal in our culture, but it is opening the door to overeating. It is very difficult to stay within your calorie guidelines while having meals spread throughout the day. This overeating leads to weight gain, heart conditions, type 2 diabetes, and more.

Intermittent fasting is here to help solve some of these issues. It works to restrict you're eating window so instead of allowing yourself to eat all day, you will only eat for a specified number of hours each day. There are also options that require you to go all day without eating. The idea here is when you restrict how much time you can eat; you can naturally restrict how many calories you consume.

In addition, intermittent fasting forces the body to delve into its fat stores in order to fuel the body through the day. Even if you are getting enough calories during the day, it is likely that the body will run out between the start of the fast and when it ends (usually sixteen hours or more for the fast). Instead of providing the body with food right away, you will make it go into the fat reserves of the body to provide you with enough energy.

This works for you in several ways. First, you still get the benefit of having enough energy, even if it has been awhile since you have eaten. None of the intermittent fasts go long enough that you are truly starving your body, so you won't have to deal with that issue.

Second, you can lose weight on an intermittent fast. When you eat fewer calories and ask the body to metabolize some of the extra fat around your body, you are going to see weight loss in no time. Even after just a few weeks, it is likely that you will be able to visibly see the differences in weight loss.

And thirdly, when you ask the body to go through all the reserve fat that is on the body, you can get rid of all that excess fat around the middle. That excess fat on your stomach and thighs is not only unattractive to most people, it can also cause a lot of health conditions. By digging into that area of your body and using it for energy, you are not only making yourself look nicer and fitter, you are also improving your health.

One nice thing about intermittent fasting is that you are the one in control. Basically, if you make sure that your eating windows are smaller than your fasting windows, you will see some results. There are several options when it comes to an intermittent fast, and you can easily choose the one that works best for your hunger levels, your comfort levels, and even with your schedule.

How Intermittent Fasting Helps Improve Insulin Sensitivity

When you take in food, your body is going to break it all down in the stomach. The glucose, or the sugar, from that food is then going to be absorbed into the bloodstream and transported to the cells. Glucose is not always a bad thing. It is there to give your cells the fuel that is needed to complete their jobs.

Insulin is the hormone that will tell your cells that they should accept the glucose fuel from the blood. When the body receives a signal that you have eaten, the beta cells in your pancreas will work to produce the insulin, which will then get to work and will tell your cells to absorb that glucose.

When the individual doesn't have this insulin, which can happen when you have diabetes, the cells are not going to allow the glucose to come in. This glucose will stay in the bloodstream. And once the body sees that the glucose has been sitting around the blood for some time, it is going to grab that glucose and store it as fat to use later because it assumes that the cells don't need the glucose right now.

When insulin comes into play and signals to the cells that fuel is coming, and the cells respond by receiving the glucose from the bloodstream, then you receive the adequate amounts of energy. When this all works properly, you are not going to pack on the body fat. But there are times when this kind of communication is going to be thrown off.

Insulin resistance is going to happen when the delivery knocks on the doors of the cells, but they don't answer. Insulin is there to signal that the food is coming, but the cells are not going to allow the glucose to come in. Instead of the cells receiving the glucose and the energy that they need, that sugar is going to stay in the bloodstream. After some time, the body recognizes this and will store that sugar as body fat.

If nobody is answering the door at first, the body is going to send more of the insulin knocking. The pancreas is going to produce more of the insulin and try to turn up the signal more to see if the cells will absorb the glucose. Sometimes this little extra insulin is enough to tell the cells how to respond. But insulin resistance can occur when the cells are stubborn, and they still won't respond to this signal.

The pancreas can only keep up with the extra production of insulin for so long. When the pancreas gets tired, you are going to end up with a variety of problems, such as diabetes, pre-diabetes, or insulin deficiency.

There are a lot of different symptoms that you may notice in someone who is insulin resistant. Often these signals can take a long time to form, which is why many people will have this problem for years before anyone will notice. Some of the signs that can come with this insulin resistance include:

- Fatigue
- Trouble with concentrating
- High blood pressure
- Fluid retention and swelling that shows up in the ankles.
- Skin tags
- Scalp hair loss in women
- Feeling hungry and angry often

- Carb and sugar cravings

- Fatty liver disease

- Polycystic ovarian syndrome

- Acne

- A fasting blood sugar level that is elevated

- Patches of dark skin over the body

- Some extra weight in the middle of the body.

The next question you may have is how can you fix this insulin resistance? The best way to make your cells more sensitive to the insulin you get is to go through a period of fasting. If you are dealing with insulin resistance, this is often because the levels of insulin in the body are often high all the time. Your body is constantly trying to shove the energy into fat cells, and this can make you feel tired and lousy.

Intermittent fasting is one of the easiest and best ways to help with this insulin resistance. Researchers have been able to measure significant results in two weeks or less, and one study has found that an intermittent fast could work better than cutting calories to help with your levels of insulin.

An intermittent fast may seem hard to get started with. You may worry that it will be hard to skip breakfast or lunch, but there are some things that you can do to make this process easier. For example, you could have a late breakfast that is full of pure fat, without a lot of carbs or protein. This could send out a signal to the body that you are not starving, without messing up the fast that you are doing.

How does intermittent fasting work to help with insulin resistance? Once your body has burnt through all the glucose that is available, it is going to move onto glycogen for energy, which is the stored glucose. After your body goes through these stores, the body can go into a small state of ketosis but will help you to burn even more fat off the body. When it is combined with the ketogenic diet, which can be a popular addition to the intermittent fast, you may be able to burn off more calories and more fat at the same time.

When you go on an intermittent fast, you are giving your body a break from all the insulin that is in the body. And often, this can help enough to make the cells more sensitive to the insulin and the glucose you eat. In addition, you will find that when you go on the fast, the body is more likely to use up some of your stored glycogen, or the glucose that has been stored as body fat, as energy, helping you to lose body fat and feel better in no time.

Intermittent Fasting and Human Growth Hormones
Human growth hormone, or HGH, is a hormone that is made by our pituitary gland. This hormone will play a big role in the normal development of children and adolescents. But it can also play a role in adults. When an adult is suffering from a deficiency in HGH, it could lead to them having higher levels of body fat, a decreased amount of bone mass, and a lower lead body mass.

Once the HGH is released from the pituitary gland, it is only able to stick around in the bloodstream for a few minutes. It will go over to the liver to be metabolized, and then it is converted into other growth factors. One of the most important of these growth factors is IGF1 or Insulin-Like Growth Factor.

This is the IGF1 that will be connected to higher levels of insulin and many other poor outcomes of your health. But the pulse that comes from IGF1 will only last a few minutes and no longer. All the hormones are going to be released naturally in short bursts to ensure that the body doesn't develop a resistance to them. This resistance can happen if there are high levels of a hormone and that hormone persists at staying at those high levels.

Growth hormone is one that will be released while the person is asleep, and it is known as a counter-regulatory hormone. Along with adrenaline and cortisol, HGH will increase your blood glucose because it helps to break down glycogen. This means that HGH can help counter the bad health effects of insulin. These hormones are going to be released shortly before you wake, usually around four in the morning, during your counter-regulatory stage. This is completely normal and the point of it is to ensure that your body is ready for the new day by pushing some of your glucose from storage so that it is in the bloodstream and ready for use as energy.

The idea that you must eat something for breakfast in order to gain enough energy to get through the morning is completely wrong. Because of the process above, your body has already provided you with the fuel that you need to get moving. You don't need to eat a ton of sugary cereal or a lot of carbs to get your energy. This burst of energy that naturally comes from the body is the reason that hunger is usually still low in the morning, even though you have gone twelve hours without eating.

One thing to note about HGH is that the levels in the body are going to go down as you get older. And if the levels get abnormally low, you could end up with lower bone and muscle mass. But couldn't we just give HGH to those who have very low levels? Let's look at a study that was done in 1990 and published in an article in New England Journal of Medicine.

The first group is the HGH group and then group two is the control group or the one that doesn't have any HGH. Over six months, the weight stayed similar in both groups, but there was a lot of change in the lean body mass of the participants who took HGH.

The group that took HGH added on 8.8 percent leaner pass. This resulted in about eight pounds of extra lean muscle mass. They also found a fat mass that was 5.3 pounds lower. Even the thickness of the skin improved in those who took the HGH.

In another article that was published in JAMA in 2002, it was found that similar results were found in women as well. But if there is so much good for those who took the HGH, why isn't this recommended for everyone who needs to gain more lean muscle or anyone who is worried about aging?

Remember that taking HGH does come with side effects. And these studies were only showing how HGH could work for those who had very low levels of HGH, not anyone who is in the normal ranges for this hormone. In addition, those who took more HGH found an increase in blood sugars, which means that the incidents of pre-diabetes in the participants grew as well. There were other side effects such as higher blood pressure and an increase in fluid retention. Over the long term, there was also a risk of increase heart problems and prostate cancer.

While HGH is a normal hormone that is released in the body, artificial injections of this hormone can prove to cause a lot of health concerns in the individual. Since this is not such a good thing, it is much better to find an all-natural method of increasing this growth hormone. And that method is to fast on a regular basis.

Kerndt et al published a study in 1982 of one patient who decided, for religious purposes, to go on a forty day fast. There were some amazing results that occurred. First, the glucose levels of the patient went down. This patient started out with a 96-glucose level and then it dropped down to 56. Insulin levels also go way down. They started at 13.5 and then dropped to 2.91 and stayed there for the remainder of the fast. As you can see, if you are worried about pre-diabetes or type 2 diabetes, then fasting may be the best solution for you to try out in order to bring down your high insulin.

But what caused this? This study also looked at the HGH levels during that time. For this patient, it started at 0.73 and then it peaked at 9.86. This is an increase of 1,250 percent for HGH. Even a short fast, perhaps one that is only five days long, could give you a huge increase, up to 300 percent. This shows that you can naturally increase your levels without having to take it artificially.

What about all those bad side effects that we talked about before, the ones that seemed to bother patients who took artificial injections of HGH? They didn't show up when the levels of HGH were increased naturally.

Other studies have shown that this increase in human growth hormone will happen when the individual goes on a fast. In 1988, HO KY et al studied fasting and how it affected HGH levels. On a control day, you could eat meals that would suppress HGH release, which is normal considering HGH will increase glucose and will be suppressed when you eat.

Fasting is one of the best ways to stimulate the release of HGH. When you fast, there is going to be a spike of this hormone early in the morning, but then there is also a regular release of it throughout the day.

This release of HGH is going to be very crucial to helping you maintain your lean bass, both with your bone mass and with muscle mass. This goes against some of the common misconceptions about fasting is that it would make you lose lean muscle mass. But studies have shown that this doesn't occur and that you will see an increase in your lean muscle mass. When compared with traditional caloric reduction diets, fasting did a much better job at preserving your lean mass, up to four times better.

This idea assumes that the body would start going through the lean muscle mass instead of the stored fat when we need energy during a fast. But this is not something the body would do. Lean muscle mass only gets used up when you reach intense starvation, a starvation that lasts for a very long time and when calories have been extremely restricted. This doesn't happen with an intermittent fast. You still get to eat, and your fasting is usually not for more than 24-hours at a time.

As a result, the body is going to burn through the extra fat stored in the body, rather than dealing with the muscle. It doesn't make a lot of sense for the body to burn through the muscle mass unless it was desperate. The muscle is needed to help the body move and function, but the fat is just sitting around. It makes more sense for the body to burn up that extra fat and that is just what the intermittent fast helps it to do.

Intermittent fasting can be a great option for those who are looking to lose weight and get their health on track. While there are a lot of people who don't understand how this fasting process works and who will spread the wrong information about it due to that, fasting has all the benefits that you have been looking for when it comes to a healthier you.

Chapter 2:
The Benefits of an Intermittent Fast

There are many different benefits to following an intermittent fast. Simply by rearranging the times you eat during the day and limiting the bad foods that you take in; you can improve your health better than ever before. Some of the benefits you can get from following an intermittent fast include:

Lose Weight

Many people go on an intermittent fast to help them lose weight. If done correctly, an intermittent fast can help you to eat fewer meals during the day. Unless you are overcompensating by eating a lot of food during your eating window, you will naturally take in fewer calories, and that alone can help with weight loss.

Additionally, intermittent fasting can enhance how your hormones function, which can aid in weight loss as well. For example, when you have naturally lower insulin levels, higher levels of human growth hormone, and an increased amount of norepinephrine, it is going to increase how much body fat is broken down and can make it easier for the body to use this fat as a source of energy.

Because of these reasons, a short-term fast could help to increase your rate of metabolism. The increase can range between 3.6 to 14 percent. When your metabolism goes faster, you can burn more calories and lose weight in the process.

This means that intermittent fasting can work on both sides of the equation. It is going to boost the rate of your metabolism, so it increases the calories that you burn, and it can reduce how much food you eat because you have a smaller eating window.

According to a study conducted in 2104, intermittent fasting can really help with weight loss. This study found that over a time period of three to twenty-four weeks, those who practiced intermittent fasting saw weight loss of three to eight percent. This is significant, especially when compared to those who only restricted their calories.

In addition, these participants also were able to lose between four and seven percent off their weight circumference. The importance of this is that it indicates they lost belly fat, a harmful fat that can cause many harmful health diseases. And another review study showed how this kind of fasting could cause less lean muscle loss compared to a diet of continuous calorie restriction.

Reduce Your Risk of Type 2 Diabetes

Type 2 diabetes has become a common problem for many people in recent years. The main feature of this kind of diabetes is high blood sugar levels because the cells are resistant to the insulin that is sending them a message. When the cells aren't listening to the insulin, they won't absorb the glucose, and it sits around in the blood stream.

Anything that you do that helps to reduce the amount of resistance your body has to insulin is going to help lower your levels of blood sugars and can do a lot for protecting you against type 2 diabetes. Intermittent fasting has been shown to have many benefits for insulin resistance and it was able to provide an impressive reduction in the levels of blood sugar in most individuals who decided to follow the fast.

In human studies, those who were on an intermittent fast found that their fasting blood sugar reduced up to six percent. But their fasting insulin levels reduced by twenty to thirty-one percent.

One study that was done on diabetic rats also showed how going on an intermittent fast could protect against damages to the kidneys, something that is a severe complication with diabetes. What this shows is that intermittent fasting may be a great choice for those who have or are at risk of developing type 2 diabetes.

However, you must be aware that there may be differences in how this works between the genders. One study that was done in women showed that control of blood sugar got worse after they followed 22 days of an intermittent fasting protocol. More studies would have to be done on this, and it may just be a factor of changing around how long you fast for women to get the same benefits as well.

Reduces Inflammation in the Body
Oxidative stress is hard on the body and it can be one of the risk factors that come with aging and other chronic diseases. This kind of stress is going to involve a lot of free radicals, or molecules that are considered unstable, reacting with some of the important molecules that your body needs. These

important molecules can be things like DNA and protein in the body. When the free radicals react with the important molecules, they will end up causing damage.

There have been several studies that show how intermittent fasting is a great way to enhance how your body resists oxidative stress. In addition, there are other studies that talk about how intermittent fasting is important for fighting off inflammation. Inflammation can be hard on the body because it is going to be the key force behind many other harmful diseases in the body. With the help of intermittent fasting, you can effectively reduce the amount of inflammation that is in the body and get your health back on track.

Can Help Improve Your Heart Health

It is important that we take care of the heart we have. We only get one. But currently, heart disease is considered one of the biggest killers throughout the world. The good news is that there are various health markers that are associated with either decreasing or increasing your risk of heart disease.

Intermittent fasting can be helpful for your heart because studies have shown how it can help improve some of the risk factors for heart disease. This includes your blood pressure, your LDL and total cholesterol, blood sugar levels, inflammatory markers, and more.

However, since intermittent fasting is still a new type of dieting and eating plan, there are not a lot of studies done on it yet. But from animal studies, and reports from those who have chosen to go on an intermittent fast, the effects on heart health seem to be positive.

May Be Able to Prevent Your Risk of Cancer

Cancer is a word that no one wants to hear. They don't want to hear that they have it, or that a loved one is dealing with it. Cancer is a disease that has uncontrolled growth of cells throughout the body and can make it hard for regular cells to grow and get the nutrients they need.

There is some research that shows that fasting can have benefits on the metabolism, including several that could reduce your risk of developing cancer during your lifetime. Although there still haven't been human studies done on this, there is promising evidence from animal studies that show how intermittent fasting may be an effective tool at preventing cancer.

In addition, fasting could also help patients who are going through chemotherapy. Chemotherapy can be hard on the body and the psychological toll can make it worse. But several studies have shown how fasting can help with chemotherapy and lesson some of the bad side effects.

Fasting Can Improve the Functioning of Your Brain
Doing something that is good for the body can often be good for your brain as well. Intermittent fasting can help improve a variety of your metabolic features, many of which are also important for the health of your brain. This could include some of the benefits that we talked about above, including reducing your blood sugar levels, reducing insulin resistance, reducing inflammation, and reducing oxidative stress.

There have been several different animal studies that show how well intermittent fasting can help increase the growth of new nerve cells. When these nerve cells grow properly and can repair themselves, it is going to provide a lot of benefits for brain function.

Intermittent fasting can also help to increase the levels of a brain-derived neurotrophic factor or BDNF. When the body has a deficiency in this, it could result in depression and some other brain problems in the individual. When you can increase this brain hormone, you could help to keep the brain stronger than ever.

In some beginning studies done on animals, it may be possible that intermittent fasting would protect against brain damage that usually comes with stroke. These are just some of the beginning studies done on intermittent fasting and how it can be so good for your brain.

Can Help to Prevent Alzheimer's Disease
If you have a family history of Alzheimer's, or you just want to be proactive and reduce your chances of developing this mental disorder, then going on an intermittent fast may be the right option for you. Alzheimer's is one of the most common neurodegenerative diseases in the world. There is no known cure for this disease right now, so it is very important that you learn how to prevent it before it even starts.

One study that was done on rats shows how an intermittent fast could help to delay the start of Alzheimer's in some patients and could even reduce how severe the disease is. in addition, a series of case reports, doing different lifestyle changes, including some daily short-term fasts, were able to help improve the symptoms of Alzheimer's in ninety percent of the patients.

Can Help Extend Your Life
Another benefit of going on an intermittent fast is that it could help you to extend your lifespan. Studies that have been done in rats show how

intermittent fasting can extend your lifespan in a manner that is like continuous calorie restriction. In some of these studies, the effects are very prominent. In one, it found that rats who fasted every other day tended to live up to 83 percent longer than the rats who didn't fast at all.

If you are looking for a way to prolong your life and to fight illnesses, then intermittent fasting may be the right choice for you. With the help of better eating habits, less stress, and less inflammation on the body, intermittent fasting can add many years to your life.

Studies have yet to show the benefits of longevity on humans who use an intermittent fast, but it does show some promising results. Intermittent fasting has become popular among the anti-aging group and it could be your key to keeping yourself young.

Chapter 3:
Common Side Effects of Intermittent Fasting

When you first get started on an intermittent fast, there are a few side effects that you will need to watch out for. The good news is that these side effects usually fade out within the first week of your fast. So, if you can make it through the first few days, you are going to be just fine on a fast, and you will see the results. Some of the side effects that you should watch out for on this fast includes:

Hunger
With a traditional American diet, you usually eat between five to six times a day. When you do this, your body learns how to expect food at certain times. Your hormone levels are going to keep with the same pattern as before, at least in the beginning, when you start with your intermittent fast. This means that even though you are on a fast, your body may feel hungry at the same times as before. This takes some willpower to get through, and usually, days three to five will feel like the worst. But over time, the hormone levels will change, and you will be able to get onto the new schedule.

To help combat the hunger that you are feeling, make sure that in the first few weeks, you drink a lot of water. This can help you to feel a bit more satisfied, can add some more alertness to the day, and can keep the belly full. A good thing to try is that within the first half hour after you wake up, try to drink at least twelve ounces of water to help. And then, any time you feel some hunger pains in your stomach, especially during the fasting time, consider drinking another 12 ounces or more.

This is one thing that an intermittent fast will help you learn. Many times, when you feel hungry, it is more that the body is bored or thirsty, rather than hungry. Give yourself some water and see if the hunger pains stick around.

Headaches

As your body gets used to this new kind of eating schedule, you may find that a few dull headaches, ones that kind of come in and out, will be normal. These will go away, but it is important to realize they may be there. Often this is caused by dehydration, which is another common issue during the fast. Make sure that you drink a lot of water during your fasting and the feeding windows to limit the headaches as much as possible.

Sometimes the headaches are going to be caused when your blood sugar levels decrease, or when stress hormones are released when you fast. With time, the body is going to get used to this eating schedule. Just try to keep stress down to a minimum and you will find this one gets better.

Low Energy

The first few days of the fast are going to be hard because you will be low on energy. Because the body isn't getting a constant source of fuel from the food like you usually do, you will feel a little bit sluggish during that first week on a fast. Try to keep the first little bit of a fast as relaxed as you can so that you don't exert a ton of energy. You may even want to keep the workouts to a minimum during this time and just do some light yoga or walking to keep active until the body can adjust.

Irritability

When you feel hungry, it can sometimes lead to you feeling angry at the same time. People who first get started on an intermittent fast will experience issues with feeling a bit grumpy any time their blood sugar levels drop, or when they are dealing with some of the other side effects. You may want to spend some of the first few days of your fast alone to avoid running into trouble with other people.

Heartburn and Bloating

During a fast, the stomach is going to produce some acid to digest food, but since you are not eating anything, that acid is just sitting there and can cause heartburn in many cases. Time is going to help with this one. As the body gets used to the different time periods you are eating now, you will get less acid in the stomach and the heartburn will go away.

Feeling Cold

Some people who go on these fasts will experience cold toes and fingers when they are on a fast. When you fast, the blood flow in the body is going to increase to the fat stores. This is known as adipose tissue blood flow, which is important because it is going to help move the fat of the body over to the muscles so that it can be burned just like fuel. This can make some people more sensitive to feeling cold.

Issues with Overeating

When it is time to stop the fast and start to eat, you will have to learn how to control yourself. The body doesn't want to go to a fast in the beginning because it is so used to being able to eat all throughout the day. You will have cravings and will want to eat right when the fast is done. But it is easy to overeat, and this can make it hard to keep within your calorie allotment. Coming up with a meal plan and having healthy options around when you do break your fast, and you will be able to safely end that fast without ruining all your hard work.

Chapter 4:
Choices for Intermittent Fasting

Now that we know a little bit more about intermittent fasting and why it is such a good thing for you to try, it is time to learn some of the different methods that are available for you to choose from when you get started on intermittent fasting. One of the nice things about intermittent fasting is that there isn't a "one size fits all" kind of mentality. There are quite a few different types of fasts that you can choose, and all of them can provide you with some results. Some of the most popular methods that you can choose from when you get started with intermittent fasting include:

The 16/8 Method

One of the most popular methods for intermittent fasting is the 16/8 method. This is where you will fast each day, for about 14 to 1 hours, and then you can eat for the remaining eight to ten hours. During this eating window, you can fit in two or three meals, if you are careful about how many calories you consume.

This method of fasting can be simple to do. For example, if you choose to wake up and not eat breakfast one day, you would be on this type of intermittent fast. You could stop eating supper at 7 pm and then wait until 11 am the next day. This is enough time for you to have fasted for 16 hours. You would just repeat this cycle each day to see the results.

One thing to note is that most of the time it's not recommended that women fast for much more than 15 hours. These shorter fasts seem to work better for them and ensure that the intermittent fast isn't going to mess with a woman's hormones and cause other issues. Fourteen to fifteen hours is plenty long enough to get the benefits of intermittent fasting without any worries for women.

For those who get hungry when they first wake up in the morning and who are used to eating breakfast, then this kind of fast can be hard for them to get used to. However, after a week or so, you will get used to the change and won't even miss breakfast anymore.

During this kind of fast, you can drink water, coffee, and any other non-caloric beverage. If you start to feel hungry during the fast, consider drinking some extra water. This will help to reduce your levels of hunger until you reach your eating window.

You should also concentrate on eating mostly healthy foods when you are not fasting. While there isn't a set diet plan that goes with intermittent fasting, you won't be able to see the results if you eat a ton of junk food or if you make up for all the calories that you missed during your eating window.

The 5:2 Diet

The 5:2 diet is another choice that you can go with. This diet involves you eating your normal diet for five days of the week, and then you will restrict your calories down to no more than 600 on two days of the week. This can be effective, if you stick with the calorie allowances and you don't have the two fasting days in a row. On the fasting days, women should stick with about 500 calories, and men should stick with 00 calories.

An example of the 5:2 diet is where you might choose to eat a normal diet on all the days of the week except Monday and Thursdays. On these days, you will choose to eat two small meals, that are between 250 and 300 calories each. This helps you to effectively reduce the number of calories that you consume each day and can give you some of the other health benefits that come with intermittent fasting.

Fat Loss Forever
This is an intermittent fast that is going to take some of the best parts of some of the other fasts and then combines them together into one new plan. You also get to have one day to cheat each week, and then that must be followed by a 36 hour fast. After that, the rest of the seven days are going to be split up between the different types of intermittent fasting.

For this one to work, you should save your longest fasts for those days when you are busy. This makes it easier for you to focus on being productive and getting things done, rather than focusing on the meals that you are missing. This type of plan can also include some training programs, so you can lose as much weight as possible.

According to the ones who started this type of intermittent fast, while everyone does do a little fasting each day, such as when you are sleeping, most people do it in a sporadic way that does make it harder to get the rewards. This program offers you a seven-day schedule of fasting so that the body can get used to this new timetable and can get the most out of the fasting periods. Plus, its ads in a cheat day that a lot of people like.

This method is specific though and since the fasting and feeding schedule changes so much during the day, some people find that it is a hard one to follow. There are tools to make this easier though.

Eat Stop Eat

With the eat stop eat fasting method, you will do a 24-hour fast, usually once or twice each week. This method has been popular for some time because it is so effective to follow. By choosing to fast from the end of dinner on one day to dinner on the next, you end up with a 24-hour fast. You can easily fit this into your schedule by choosing the busiest day of the week and making that the day you fast.

An example of the eat stop eat is if you finish dinner at 7 pm on Monday. You would go to bed and then skip breakfast and lunch, along with any regular snacks, for the rest of that day. Then at 7 pm on Tuesday, you could have dinner and end the fast. You can choose to do this from any meal you choose. Going from lunch to lunch or breakfast to breakfast can be efficient to.

During this fasting time, you can have coffee, water, and other non-caloric beverages, but no solid food is allowed. If you are trying to lose weight with the eat stop eat method, then you must make sure that you eat in a normal way during all your eating periods. This means, choose to eat the same amount of food that you would if you hadn't been fasting. Don't binge and take in all the calories that you missed, or you will never lose weight.

The biggest issue with this method is that it can be hard for a lot of people to go on a 24 hour fast. However, you can build up to this. Perhaps try one of the other methods first, such as the 16/8 method, and get used to fasting. You can then build up to missing out on eating for a whole day.

Alternate Day Fasting

You can also choose to go with the alternate day fast. This means that you will go on a fast every other day of the week. There are different options that come with this, so it is going to depend on which one you like the most. Some versions will allow you to eat a little bit on your fasting day, but you usually need to keep the calories for that day under 600.

Many lab studies that show how healthy intermittent fasting can be used some version of the alternate day fast. This means that if you want to get the health benefits from intermittent fasting, then this may be the one you want to choose. However, having a full day fast every other day can seem extreme, so you may want to build up to this.

One thing to remember is that you don't have to wake up in the morning and start your fast from there. This would technically put you at a 36 hour or so fast. Instead, after you are done with supper one day, start the clock. You can then eat on the next day at supper time again. This can make it a bit easier to stick with the alternate day fast.

The Warrior Diet

Another option that you can choose to try is known as the Warrior Diet. This intermittent fast is going to involve you eating just small amounts of vegetables and raw fruits throughout the day. Then at night, you can eat one big meal. Basically, you will be fasting all day, and then you can spend four hours at night feasting.

With the Warrior Diet, you will only eat for four hours during the day. You can technically eat however much you want during those four hours. But since it is such a small window of time to eat, it is unlikely that you will go over your calorie allowance in that time frame.

For the other twenty hours of the day, you will focus on fasting. You can have minimal amounts of fresh fruits and vegetables to help keep the metabolism running and to ensure that you aren't too hungry, but most of your calories during the day must come during that four-hour period.

In addition, the Warrior Diet is often going to emphasize foods that are like what is found on the paleo diet. This means that if you choose the Warrior Diet, you will stick with foods that are unprocessed and whole, and ones that look like they come from nature.

This version of an intermittent fast can be hard to stick with. It only allows you to eat for four hours during the day. Yes, you can graze a little on fruits and vegetables before this four-hour window if you choose, but the amount that you eat during those times must be minimal. This is the method chosen for those who are trying to see results very quickly, such as those who need to lose a lot of weight or those trying to get ready for strength training competitions.

Bulletproof Intermittent Fasting

Bulletproof intermittent fasting is a bit different compared to some of the other forms of fasting we have talked about. It is there to let you fast for a longer time without feeling hungry while also building muscle and get rid of fat at the same time.

With this method, you will go on a fast, such as the 16/8 fast, but in the morning, you can make one change. With this method, you will have a cup of bulletproof coffee at some point in the morning. This does technically break the fast, but you will only have that coffee, and nothing else, until later in the day. Then you would enjoy two regular sized meals later in the day before starting the fast again.

The Bulletproof coffee is meant to make all the difference. This coffee is special because it contains a lot of healthy fats from grass-fed butter and brain octane oil. These ingredients will work together to give you a stable current of energy to sustain you through the day. Even though there aren't a ton of calories in the coffee, it has enough other nutrients to keep you full, and it's possible that you would be able to make it through quite a few hours before you needed to eat anything at all.

The Master Cleanse

Another option that you can choose when looking for a fast is the Master Cleanse. This one is sometimes known as the lemonade diet as well. This is one that many celebrities have gone on to lose weight, but since it doesn't really include a lot of healthy eating principles, the results are probably not going to stick around for a long time.

This diet plan is known as a liquid-only diet that includes three different things. It has a lemonade like beverage, an herbal laxative tea, and a saltwater drink. The claim with this one is simple. It states that if you give this diet at least ten days, you can drop a lot of weight, detox out the digestive system, and feel healthy, energetic, and happy. It also states that the cleanse is a good way to curb some of your cravings for those unhealthy foods that you are stuck on.

The next question you may have is how does the Master Cleanse work. Because you are relying on this lemonade drink, you are not taking in a lot of calories. This lack of calories can cause you to lose weight. However, it's likely that you would lose a lot of water weight as well. And since it is not a sustainable method to work with, it is sometimes seen as a method that is going to put the weight right back on when you're done. However, if you are looking for a way to break some of your bad eating habits before using a different intermittent fast, then this is a good option to try.

When you follow his kind of cleanse, the only thing that you can have is an herbal laxative tea and a salt-water lemonade drink. You are not allowed to have any solid food, and alcohol is out of the question while you are on this diet. This is the diet that is recommended for ten days.

After the ten days are done, it is fine to start adding in some other foods, if you do it slowly. You would start with soup and juice, and then lead yourself over to raw vegetables and fruits. If you want to keep with the Master Cleanse, you will probably need to stick with a more vegetarian diet because it recommends that you eat very little meat and that you stay away from dairy products.

This is a very hard diet to follow. You are essentially relying on a liquid diet for ten days, and that can be hard. It is likely that you are going to feel hungry often and you may have to deal with side effects like headaches, boredom, tiredness, and cravings. And this cleanse claims that you need to follow this diet exactly, or you will not see the results.

Most people who go on this cleanse will make some modifications. For example, they may stick with the liquid diet for most of the day, but then they will allow themselves to have a meal at the end of the day, perhaps with some fish and healthy fruits and vegetables. This allows them to get some nutrition in without having to lose all the benefits of the cleanse.

Spontaneous Meal Skipping

One thing that you will notice when you go on an intermittent fast is that it's not necessary to follow a rigid and structured fasting plan in order to get some of the benefits from this eating plan. You can still get some of the benefits if you only skip meals from time to time. If there is a day when you are too busy to eat or cook, or if there is a time when you just don't feel hungry, then skip that meal and eat later when you are hungry.

While the American culture believes that you need to eat every few hours and have all those meals every day, or you will hit starvation mode, this is not true. The human body is designed to handle long periods of famine, such as what would happen when our ancestors went through a time with little food. Missing out on a few meals here and there is not that big of a deal. Our bodies can handle it. It only becomes a problem if you miss out on most of your meals most of the time.

So, if you find that you are not that hungry one day, go ahead and skip breakfast. You can choose to eat a healthy dinner or lunch at another time. If you are traveling and don't like your food options, do a short fast. If you have a day where you are particularly busy and just can't find the time to stop and eat, then just skip a meal or two. Skipping a meal when you feel inclined is the basis of a spontaneous meal skipping fast. Just double check that you are eating plenty of healthy foods at the other meals you choose.

As you can see, there are many different choices out there for an intermittent fast. You can go with the option that works the best for your needs. Some people find that just having a mini fast during each day works the best to put them on a schedule, and others like the ability to go on a full day fast when they are busy. You can pick any of these fasts and still get amazing results.

Chapter 5:
Starving Yourself Vs Intermittent Fasting

One common misconception about intermittent fasting is that it is going to make you go into starvation mode. We have been taught that missing one meal, much less going on a fast for a whole day, could put us into starvation mode, make it impossible to lose weight, and can even take away lean muscle mass. All this misinformation, and it is no wonder that people are hesitant about starting an intermittent fast.

Fasting and starvation are similar in that they require the individual to abstain from food. The main differences between these two are the length of time and the purpose of that abstinence. In both cases, the psychological changes that take place are going to help the body adapt to the deficiency of nutrients that are present. While fasting for the short-term can be a safe thing to do, if you prolong it by too much, it can become harmful.

The Source of Fuel for the Body
When you eat a meal, the body is going to take that food and break it down into amino acids, fatty acids, and sugars. These are important because they are the basic building blocks that are needed to maintain the processes of the body.

Sugar, also known as glucose, when it gets into the body, is going to be used by the cells as a form of energy. If the cells do not use all the glucose that you eat, then it is going to be changed to glycogen and then stored in the muscles and the liver of the body. Fat is another important building block of the food you consume. Fat will often be stored as fatty acids, and you can find them in the adipose tissue of the body. These are also known as the fat cells of the body. And finally, amino acids are found in the food as well. Amino acids are the protein that is so important to building up the muscles.

If you go for some time without eating food, then you are not consuming these important nutrients. But the body still needs them during this time of not eating. The body is going to resort to metabolizing the stored fat, glycogen, and muscle protein in order to meet its nutritional needs during this time.

Starving vs. Fasting

The process above is going to occur no matter whether you are starving yourself or you are fasting. But if you abstain from food for too long, there could be some more issues that come up.

When you are not taking in food, there are some hormonal changes that occur in the body. These changes are important because they allow the body to use up its stored nutrients. For example, glucagon, epinephrine, and insulin are all hormones that are going to help regulate the levels of blood sugar in the body. Insulin is going to help you bring down blood sugar levels because it causes the cells to take up glucose. Epinephrine and glucagon are important parts here because they are going to elevate blood sugars by controlling how glycogen breaks down.

During starvation, you will see something else happen. Insulin is going to decrease, while epinephrine and glucagon are going to increase. Therefore, you are going to feel hungry. The interplay between these hormones will ensure that you are able to keep your levels of blood sugars stable during a fast. This is a good thing when you are fasting.

But when you reach the level of starvation, glycogen is all used up and molecules known as ketones are going to be created from stored fatty acids. This happens so that you have an alternative fuel to keep the body moving. Once the body has used up all that fat and the ketones, it is going to move on to the protein from the muscles in order to make glucose as well.

With fasting, you are abstaining from food for a short amount of time. You are just going to miss out on a few hours of eating at a time. This results in a positive change in the hormones in your body which will provide you with a way to burn off the extra fat that is stored in the body. You will go back to a regular pattern of eating long before the body gets to use up all the glycogen, fat, and then moves on to the muscles for fuel.

With starvation, you have gone on a fast for a very long time. Instead of spending 24-hours or less on a fast, you have probably severely limited your calories for weeks if not longer. The body is not receiving the food and nutrients that it needs to function, plus it has gone through all the reserved energy in the body. This is when food avoidance is going to be dangerous on the body. When your body must resort to breaking down its own muscles for protein, you will see a host of issues, such as the distortion of cells and possible organ failure and death if it goes on long enough.

To summarize, fasting is usually only going to last for a day, sometimes a little longer if you are sick. Then you will go back to your regular eating habits.

It is just long enough to use up the nutrients from the foods you ate before the fast and to maybe use some of the stored glycogen that is in the body. It is nowhere near long enough to cause permanent damage and can be good for the body.

With starvation, you have taken your food abstinence too far. You have deprived the body of nutrients so badly, that it is resorting to using up protein from the muscles just to keep you alive. This is not a problem with fasting because the intermittent fast is not long enough. A few hours up to a few days will not cause starvation.

Reasons to Abstain from Food

Fasting and starvation are going to have very different purposes. Starvation is often the result of either an eating disorder or it could be what happens when a famine goes on and you don't have access to food. Fasting, on the other hand, is typically performed for a defined period for a specific purpose. This could be as part of a cleanse, to prepare for a medical procedure, or because of a religious practice.

Fasting is often going to include a diet that is lower in calories to help promote your health. You will substitute some of your regular eating habits to eating healthier along with the intermittent fast to help see how your health can improve. As we have already discussed, there are a ton of great health benefits that you can get from going on an intermittent fast.

Both practices are very different from each other. A small fast, either on occasion or on a regular basis, can be good for your health and can improve so many different parts of your life. But starvation can be hard on the body, whether it is intentional or not. They are two different ideas and you can safely go on a fast without worrying about the harmful issues that can come with a long-term starvation.

How to Be Safe on A Fast

There are many reasons why you may choose to go on an intermittent fast. You may want to increase your heart health, reduce risks of cancer and diabetes, or even lose weight. But when you decide to get started on a fast, you may be worried that you are going to enter starvation mode and cause harm to your body.

The first thing to realize is that it is hard for the body to go into starvation mode. Going on a fast for a day, or a few hours is not going to do it. Especially if you are careful to eat a well-balanced diet before you go on the fast. This gives the body plenty of nutrients to burn through as fuel, so you won't have to worry about the negative effects of starvation.

There is a lot of research out there to prove that a short fast is not going to cause you harm from starvation. In fact, many of us go on a short fast while we are sleeping without even realizing it. According to the American Cancer Society, fasting for a short amount of time is not likely to be harmful to the body, as long as you eat a good diet before you go on the fast, and you make sure that you take in enough fluids during the fast.

The good news is that you can go on an intermittent fast and rest easy knowing that it is healthy and safe for the body. Because the time of abstaining from food is so short, you can burn through some of the extra glycogen and stored fat in the body, without getting anywhere near the issues of starvation.

Chapter 6:
What Foods Should I Eat on An Intermittent Fast?

The next question that you may have about going on an intermittent fast is what you should choose to eat on that fast. This often depends on your personal goals and whether you plan to add a specific diet plan to the mix while you complete the fast.

Technically, when you go on an intermittent fast, there isn't a specific diet plan that is set up with it. This means that there really isn't a protocol for what you should and should not eat. With, you are never going to get the health and weight loss benefits that you want out of this fast if you only eat junk and processed foods. It doesn't matter how short you make your eating window; you just want to see the results.

When you go on an intermittent fast, you need to stick with a diet that is well-balanced. If you get in the right amount of nutrients and you keep your calories at a reasonable level, you will be happy with the results you see on this type of fast.

Many people choose to add diet plan to the mix when they are on an intermittent fast. This helps them to stick with the fast, to restrict their calories so they don't end up eating too much during their non-fasting time, and to help them see better results. The type of diet plan that you choose is completely up to personal preference.

There are different diet plans you can choose to go with on your intermittent fast. Options like the DASH diet, which is good for reducing high blood pressure, and the Mediterranean diet, which can help with weight loss, are great options. One of the most popular diet plans to go along with an intermittent fast is the ketogenic diet.

We will discuss some of the different foods that you should eat when you are fasting and on the ketogenic diet. The ketogenic diet is so popular because it enhances the benefits that you see with the fast, and it is easy to follow. When you combine the fasting with the ketogenic diet, you will be amazed at some of the results that you see.

Let's look at some of the tips that you can follow when you are trying to follow an intermittent fast and you want to make sure that you are eating the right types of foods. These rules are not hard and fast and if you take the time to eat foods that are high in nutrition and healthy, you are going to see that the intermittent fast is effective.

Foods to Eat on an Intermittent Fast
Picking out the right foods to eat when you are on an intermittent fast can be very important. You want to make sure that you are picking out foods that are healthy for you, foods that will give you the most nutrition possible since you are limiting you're eating window, and foods that will fill you up so your grumbly stomach doesn't ruin your plans during the fasting period.

Sticking with a well-balanced diet can be very important when you are on this kind of fast. It can meet all the criteria above, while also ensuring that you see the best health benefits and weight loss possible on this diet plan. But what does it mean to eat a well-balanced diet?

First, make sure that you get plenty of fruits and vegetables into the diet plan. Try to get a variety of these, rather than sticking with just one type. This helps you to get in as many nutrients to your diet as possible. A colorful plate is the best option because it ensures that you will fill up the body, without a ton of calories, and makes it easy for you to tell that you are getting in as much nutrition as you can each meal.

Next on the list is plenty of protein. Your muscles are going to be growing during the intermittent fast thanks to the increase in human growth hormone that is introduced. This means that the muscles will need some high-quality protein to help keep them strong. Many sources of protein also contain some of the good fats that you need (we will talk more about that in a moment), to help you keep your metabolism going fast. Pick out options such as chicken, ground beef, turkey, and fish for the best results.

Whole grains are also allowed on an intermittent fast. If you do decide to add the ketogenic diet to your intermittent fast, you may have to cut back on these a bit though. But for a regular intermittent fast, you can eat whole grains. This includes bread, pasta, and more. Stay away from the white and processed versions of these foods though. They may look similar, but the white versions are full of sugars and bad carbs that can make it hard to lose weight on your intermittent fast.

Fats are your friend on an intermittent fast, especially if you add in a specific diet plan to the mix, such as the ketogenic diet or the paleo diet. And if you consume the right fats, such as those in olive oil and those found in fish, you are helping your body absorb nutrients and stay full for longer.

Milk and other dairy products are kind of a touchy subject for some people. They are allowed on an intermittent fast and can be a great source of calcium and other nutrients for the body. You can choose from a variety of options, like milk, yogurt, cheese, cottage cheese, sour cream, and more. For some people though, these dairy products can cause digestive issues that make them uncomfortable. If this is the case for you, it may be a good idea to avoid dairy products while on this eating plan.

On occasion, it is fine to add in something sweet, or something that is considered a treat. We will talk in the next section about some of the foods that are not recommended on an intermittent fast because they aren't necessarily a part of a well-balanced diet plan. But, if you eat these sparingly and make sure that they don't become most of the foods you eat, then it is fine to have them on occasion.

This means that there is nothing wrong with having a candy bar on occasion or going out to eat with friends and family when you are on this eating regimen. Just make sure that you don't overdo it and that you stick to healthy foods as much as possible.

Foods to Avoid on an Intermittent Fast

When you are on an intermittent fast, you do need to pay some attention to the types of foods you are eating. No, there isn't an official diet that goes with the intermittent fast and you can have some freedom here, you will not reach your health and weight loss goals if you spend your eating window consuming sodas, baked good, processed foods, and other junk foods that are high in calories and low in nutrition.

On an intermittent fast, you should concentrate on eating a healthy diet, one that has a lot of nutrients to help promote the good health that you are looking for. This means all the bad stuff must go. First, kick out that sugar habit. It is fine to have some sugar on occasion, but it should not be the main staple in your diet. Cut out the baked goods, the sodas, the ice cream, and the white bread. These have high amounts of sugar that can make it hard to do well with your intermittent fast.

You should also be careful of processed foods. These are the ones that you will find in the freezer section of your grocery store. They may seem easy to make and they may taste good, but the number of bad fats, carbs, salts, and calories will easily put you over your daily requirements and can leave you feeling extra hungry when you are fasting. If you are looking to make meals that are quick and won't leave you in the kitchen all day, consider looking up some meals for your slow cooker or for the instant pot to get these meals done.

While on the intermittent fast, you should also try to avoid eating out as much as possible. Having something from your favorite fast food restaurant on occasion is not a bad thing. But many Americans eat out two or three, and sometimes more, times a week. This can add a lot of calories to your diet, and these foods are not that filling. Try to stay away from these fast foods (no matter how hard it is), as much as you can.

The Ketogenic Diet and Intermittent Fasting

Many people who go on an intermittent fast will also choose to follow the ketogenic diet. They often claim that this will help them to lose more weight quickly, and you can get all the health benefits of both at once. This is also a good way to ensure that you are going to eat healthy and whole foods, rather than binging or eating a lot of junk food once your fast is over.

Both an intermittent fast and the ketogenic diet have been shown to make your workouts more effective, decrease your food cravings, improve the insulin sensitivity in your body, and even balance the levels of glucose that are in the blood. All of these are very important if you are trying to achieve a sustainable weight loss and be healthier overall.

Because both diet plans have a lot of the same benefits, many have decided to combine them together to get the most benefits. If you are considering combining your intermittent fast with the ketogenic diet, we are going to discuss a few of the things that you should consider.

Because of how popular it is, there are a lot of people who have tried out the ketogenic diet. This is a diet that will have you really restrict how many carbs you consume so that your body will start to burn the stored fat, instead of carbs, for energy.

On its own, the ketogenic diet can help you to speed up your weight loss and does an amazing job at controlling cravings, which can be so important when you are ending a fast or trying to lose weight. But when you combine it together with an intermittent fast, you may be able to lose weight even faster than before, while also increasing your health.

It is possible to go on an intermittent fast without restricting your calories. This isn't the point of the fast. Rather, this fast is just going to limit the amount of time that you can eat during a specific period. Most of the time you will choose to fast between 15 to 24 hours a day. Then, when this time period is done, you can begin you're eating window.

If you combine the intermittent fast with the ketogenic diet, you can then spend your eating time consuming any amount of zero or low carb foods that you want. But you must remember that you should eat to satiety, rather than overeating. But the low carb content found in the ketogenic diet usually means that overeating is not as big of an issue as other types of foods. This can make the intermittent fast more effective.

There are several benefits of following a ketogenic diet while also on an intermittent fast. Some of these benefits include:

- Get into ketosis faster: When you enter ketosis, your body relies on the stored fat, as well as the fat in your food, to have energy, rather than relying on carbs.

- Stable your blood sugar levels.

- Better mineral and vitamin absorption: The healthy fats that you consume will help your body absorb more of the nutrients that you take in.

- Faster weight loss: both plans can help you to lose a lot of weight. When you combine both together, you will see a lot of weight loss, much more than before.

- Satisfaction: The ketogenic diet can help to curb cravings and overeating that can happen on an intermittent fast.

Eating on the ketogenic diet is a little bit different than what you would do with a traditional diet, even one that may seem healthy. The ketogenic diet is going to focus mostly on eating foods that are low in carbs, moderate in protein, and high in fats. This means that options like bread and pastas are kicked out, and even eating fruits and vegetables needs to be monitored.

The point of these foods is to ensure that your body can move over to fats and will rely on those as a form of energy, rather than relying on the carbs like we traditionally do. This helps us to feel fuller and more satisfied, can reduce cravings, and can melt off that extra fat all around the body. Some of the foods that are especially important to the ketogenic diet include:

- Seafood
- Low-carb vegetables
- Cheese
- Avocados
- Lots of poultry and meat
- Eggs
- Coconut oil
- Olive oil
- Nuts and seeds
- Plain Greek yogurt and some cottage cheese
- Berries

- Butter and cream
- Shirataki noodles
- Olives
- Unsweetened tea and coffee
- Cocoa powder and chocolate

These are a few of the things that you can consider when it comes to an intermittent fast. You can technically choose to eat anything that you would like while you are on this type of fast. But if you really want to get all the health benefits from the fast, and you really want to see weight loss, then you need to reduce the number of calories that you eat, along with the number of processed foods. Whole and nutrient dense foods will fill you up, make the fasting easier, and can ensure you get the best results possible with your choice of intermittent fast.

Chapter 7:
The Safe Way to End Your Fast

Getting on a fast is the easy part. You just finish your last meal and then don't eat until the fast is done. If you don't eat during that time period and you drink plenty of fluids, you don't have to remember too many things. But coming out of the fast in a safe manner, and in a way that isn't going to undo all the hard work you put in, can be the challenge.

When you come out of a fast, it is important to slowly ease the body back into eating regular foods. You do not want to come out of the fast and start binge eating. Sure, you will have a lot of cravings to deal with after the fast but eating too much is going to overload the digestive system and can make you feel sick in the process.

During the fast, the digestive system went through some changes. It most likely chose to reduce how many enzymes it produced because it didn't have any food to digest. This can also affect some of the mucus lining in your stomach. When you overeat or you consume foods to quickly, it could cause a lot of health concerns, like a stomachache or nausea. Plus, it can make you eat overeat and take in more calories than you should, which can make you lose out on the weight loss portion of the intermittent fast.

The key here is to introduce your regular foods back into the day slowly and strategically. This helps you to break the fast and get some food into you but also ensures that you aren't disrupting the digestive system in the process. Let's look at a strategy you can utilize that can help you safely end your fast, whether it is a full day one or not, so you can get the most benefits out of your intermittent fast.

Breaking the Fast on the First Day

The first day of the fast is often the hardest. Your body is not used to going for such a long time without food, and you are probably really feeling the hunger pains. At this point, you are ready to dive into something that is high calorie and going to fill you up quickly, even if that is not part of your dieting plan. It is so important to have a good strategy in place to help you during those first few days on the fast.

The first thing you need to do is set a timeline that is based on how long you have been fasting. This helps you to know the time frame for breaking off from the fast. Most often, it is best to have the length of your fast determine how long you will spend breaking the fast. You do not want to skip the initial breaking of the fast unless you want to deal with feeling sick. Some of the general rules that you can follow with breaking the fast include:

For a longer fast (up to seven days, though that is not recommended for an intermittent fast), you will need to set aside four days for breaking the fast. The first few days are going to be limited. You want to eat bland foods that don't have a lot of calories to help you get used to eating again.

For a one day fast, you will need to slowly start eating again. You maybe will pick out a lighter breakfast, something that can get rid of the hunger pains, but not something that is so thick and rich that it will hurt the stomach. You can have a little snack and then build up to a larger meal later in the day.

Breaking a fast can be a hard thing to do. You are going to feel ready to eat a lot of food, but if you go crazy with eating, then you are going to lose out on the weight loss benefits. And this can also end up causing some harm to your digestive tract because it isn't ready to take on that much food at once after a fast. Being careful with what you eat and taking it slowly can make all the difference as well.

Making a Meal Plan
You may find that having a meal plan in place ahead of the fast can make a big difference. This helps you to know exactly what you will eat at each point of the fast and can ensure that you won't go crazy with your eating habits in the process.

Many times, the biggest struggle after a fast is figuring out what you should eat when the fast is done. You may have some of the best intentions at the beginning, but after going a long time without eating, especially in the beginning, you are going to be hungry in the end. You may not think about the healthy meals that you could enjoy, and rather, you are probably thinking of something salty, full of fat, full of carbs, or something that is going to derail all your hard work from fasting.

With a meal plan, you can know exactly what you are going to eat at the different stages of the fast. You can plan out a whole week of meals so that you know what to eat on your fasting days (if you pick days where you can have up to the 600 calories), what you will eat when the fast is done, and what you can eat throughout your non-fasting time.

This meal plan is going to take some of the guesswork and worry out of eating after a fast and can make breaking that fast easier than before. You just need to make sure that you pick out meals that are full of great nutrients, so your body still has what it needs to stay healthy and happy, whether you are fasting or in your non-fasting time.

Other Things to Consider When on a Fast
You do need to take some care when you break a fast. It is never a good idea to eat whatever is in front of you, and as much of it as you want, right after a fast. It doesn't matter how long the fast was, eating in this manner can really harm the body. One of the best benefits of fasting can be when you realize that you broke the fast in the proper manner. Taking it slow and easy is not only a kind thing to do to the body, but it can also help you make sure that you keep your calorie count in line during this time.

If you do end up fasting for more than one day, such as getting sick during the fast or going with some of the other plans that ask for a longer fast, a good rule of thumb to remember is to take half the number of days fasted to help with the breaking. So, a fast that lasts two days would need a day to reintroduce the food to the body.

The first step here is to think about which foods you would like to eat in order to break your fast. You do not want to go for the pasta or the beads or something that is too thick and hard to digest. Sure, these may sound good and you may be craving them, but the enzymes in your body are not ready to digest these after a fast. You want to stick with foods that have lots of nutrition but are easy to digest in the beginning.

The type of fasting that you do is sometimes going to help you determine the foods that you will use in order to break the fast. While fruit and juice can be good when you are trying to break out of a water fast, they obviously aren't going to be very helpful when trying to break a fruit or a juice fast.

To help you figure out the best times to introduce different food groups, you can rely on the list below. It is going to start out with the ones that are the easiest to digest and then it will progress to the foods that can be good for you, but which should be added to the diet a little later on when the body has time to prepare for them.

Depending on how long your fast lasts, you may need to vary the amount of time that it takes to go through the list. For most intermittent fasts, you can go through this list in one day, if you take it slowly and make sure the body can handle it. And remember, it is not a requirement that you eat everything that is on this list. This is just a general list to help you know where you should be after breaking a fast. The list of foods, in order, that you can consume after a fast include:

- Vegetable and fruit juices
- Raw fruit
- Bone broths or vegetable broths
- Yogurt, without any sweeteners
- Spinach and lettuce
- Cooked vegetables as well as some vegetable soups
- Raw vegetables

- Beans and grains if they are well cooked

- Eggs and nuts

- Milk products

- Everything else

Any of the first three are great for breaking your fast. Maybe consider having some raw fruit as a little snack when you break the fast before moving on to eating something a bit heartier.

With intermittent fasting, you are usually not putting your body through a long enough fast that eating heavy foods are going to be a big deal. You should still take caution. It can be hard to stick with your calorie amounts when you are on a fast because you are so hungry. If you just dive right in, without listening to your body and seeing what happens, you are going to end up taking in too many calories and making yourself uncomfortable.

More Points to Help You Effectively Break Your Fast
There are a lot of different things that you can do to help break your fast. The method you choose is going to depend on how well your body reacts after the fast and how well you can control your hunger and your cravings. Some of the things that you can try to help make breaking the fast a little bit easier include the following:

Pay attention to how your body reacts after a fast. See if any of the foods that you eat makes you have an adverse reaction. This could be a sign that you are eating the wrong foods to break the fast, or that you may have a mild allergy to the food. Learn how to feel for the sensation of being full and then make sure that you stop eating when you reach it. You need to learn when the body is full and nourished and not just to eat when you feel a little hungry.

When you are ready to break your fast, start with a few small meals, or small snacks. After a few hours of doing this and getting the stomach adjusted, you can then progress yourself to some of the larger meals. You will be able to eat these larger meals; you just need to make sure they are not all right in the beginning.

Make sure that you are chewing your food well after a fast. This can be a good habit to foster, and it will help with proper digestion after the fast as well.

Strive to add in some good bacteria and some enzymes to the system. Fresh and raw foods are full of these enzymes that can be amazing for digestion and for your body. Probiotics, or the good bacteria, are found in pill form as well as in miso, sauerkraut, and yogurt.

While it does take a little bit of your time and attention, breaking a fast in the proper way is very important to your overall health. Plus, it is going to make it easier to lose weight and see the other health benefits that can come with intermittent fasting.

Chapter 8:
The Safe Way to Eat During Your Eating Window

Breaking the fast can be an important part of an intermittent fast. But you also need to make sure that you are careful about what you eat during the rest of your eating window. You want to make sure that you stick with your chosen diet plan, that you don't take in too many calories in the process, or you are going to miss out on some of the weight loss of this fast.

It is hard to go on a fast when you first get started. You are going to feel hungry and will want to eat everything in sight to get rid of those cravings. But if you can make it through the first few weeks of the intermittent fast, then it does get a lot easier to get through.

How Many Meals Should I have?
The next question that you may have is how many meals you should consume a day on an intermittent fast. This is often going to depend on the type of fast that you choose. For example, if you are on the Warrior Diet, you may only have time for a snack and one big meal. If you are going for a 24-hour fast, you will only have time for one meal (if you go from supper one day to supper another). But if you do the Leangains diet, you may have enough time to fit three meals in, with one smaller and two medium sized.

Often, the amount of meals you eat during the day is going to vary based on how you want to split up your calories and how much time you are giving yourself during the eating window and how hungry you are. There are no rules though, for having to eat three meals during your eating window. If that works the best for you to stick with three smaller meals, then that is a good choice.

But part of an intermittent fast is to learn how to listen to your body and eat when you are hungry or when you need to eat, not just when the time on the clock tells you it is time to eat. When you are hungry, you can eat during the eating window. When you are not, regardless of the time, then you wait.

Now, there are different thoughts out there on when you should eat. Many people ask how many meals they should eat a day to be ideal, and there are a lot of different answers for you to choose. But if you are looking to increase your lifespan and decrease your likelihood of developing many degenerative diseases, then sticking with the three-square meals each day with some snacks in between can be determinantal to this goal.

There is now growing evidence that following the three meals a day with snacks advice can be the reason that there is such an epidemic for diabetes and obesity. This is because the biggest risk of making your meals span throughout the whole day is that you are giving yourself way too many chances to overeat. This could then lead to issues with diminished health, lots of weight gain, and even metabolic dysfunction.

In the past, our ancestors were not able to get ahold of food all the time as we can today. From a historical perspective, intermittent fasting makes sense and would work well for how our bodies were designed.

According to some research done by Dr. Valter Longo, the fewer meals that you eat through the day, the better off you are going to fail. He believes that the traditional grazing approach that most Americans follow is flawed in many ways because they are only going to look at some of the short-term effects of increasing how many meals you eat each day. Yes, in the beginning doing this kind of eating pattern can help your blood sugar levels, metabolism, and appetite. But after a few months, this new system is going to find your body adapting to it. When this happens, the body is going to start craving and expecting food all the time, rather than just at mealtimes.

Modern beliefs state that it is better to just stick with two meals during the day, and maybe a little snack to help if you have a day when you are hungry. You can choose which meal that you skip though. It is often recommended that you skip out on breakfast and simply maintain the fast that you are already in. Instead of waking up and eating right away, you will extend out the fast by a few more hours, and have lunch be the first meal of the day.

This can be effective for a lot of people, but for others, it can be hard to follow. Some people are too hungry in the mornings or like breakfast too much, that they are not able to stick with this kind of diet plan. If this describes you, it may be best to skip out on dinner instead. You can then enjoy a good breakfast and lunch and cut out on your dinner so you can still follow the two meal a day rule on intermittent fasting.

The key here is to keep your eating window between six to eight consecutive hours each day. You should also avoid food for a minimum of three hours before you go to bed. Even if you decide that breakfast is the meal that you will skip, make sure that supper is early enough that you are not eating too close to bedtime at night.

The number of meals that you consume on an intermittent fast will also depend on your personal preferences, although a lot of people like the idea of going with just two meals a day. This helps them to keep from grazing through the day and can help effectively reduce the number of calories that you consume. Just make sure that the meals you are eating has plenty of healthy carbs, fats, and proteins so the body gets the fuel that it needs, and you feel full and satisfied, even during the fasting time.

How Many Calories are Recommended?

Another question that many people ask while on an intermittent fast is how many calories they should consume a day. This is going to depend on your goals. If you are on an intermittent fast for the health benefits, you may be able to eat a few more calories compared to those who are on an intermittent fast to lose weight.

If you are going on this kind of diet plan, though, you will want to make sure that you are eating the right number of calories. Remember that while intermittent fasting can do a lot of things for you, there isn't really something that is magical about it or anything that will make it possible to eat a ton of extra calories and still lose weight. Just like with other forms of dieting, you will still need to control your calories.

The good news is that since you are limiting, you're eating window with the help of intermittent fasting, you will feel like you are eating more than before, and you will feel less deprived. This is because you are putting all those calories into a smaller time period during the day, rather than relying on being able to limit your calories through the whole day. This can make it easier for you to eat healthily and stick with your calorie goals on an intermittent fast.

The first thing that you must do when it comes to figuring out how many calories you need to have on an intermittent fast is to figure out your basal metabolic rate. This is basically the number of calories that you need to eat during the day, just to stay alive. Your brain, your heart, and other important organs in the body will need to burn up some calories just to function, even if you do nothing else besides sitting on the couch.

For most individuals, this basal metabolic rate is going to be around ten to eleven calories for every pound of body weight on you. If your body has a lot of extra body fat on it, then this amount may be a little bit lower. This is still a good rule of thumb to go with and it is where we are going to start.

So, to figure out your basal metabolic rate, or the base number of calories you need, you will just take your body weight. Then multiply that number by 10 if you are a woman, or 11 for a man. Write this number down somewhere to help you out.

The next thing we are going to look for is what is known as the thermic effect of food. This is going to be the calories that the body is going to burn because you ate something. Since protein often has the highest level of thermic effect, meaning that you will burn off the most calories as the body tries to break it done, you will have a higher rate here if you eat a lot of protein. Therefore, a lot of people recommend eating more protein in their diets when they are trying to lose weight.

The number that most people will use here is 1.2. If you are on a high protein diet, you may need to add a small amount to this to see some results, but for most people, the 1.2 will be enough. To see where your calories are now, take the 1.2 and multiply it by your basal metabolic rate that we got above.

The third thing that we need to look for is our activity level. Those who tend to do more activity throughout their days are the ones who will burn up more calories throughout the day. If you have a desk job and don't move around all that much, then you will not burn up as many calories.

When figuring out this number, you need to make sure that you really are honest with yourself. If you spend most of the day at your desk and then come home and watch television most of the evening, you do not want to give yourself a score that includes workouts. You need to be honest, or you will end up with too many calories and you will not lose any weight.

The guideline that you can use to figure out how many calories you burn through the activity you do each day includes:

- A desk job should have several 1.1

- A desk job along with three workouts each week will get a 1.2

- A desk job that has at least four or five workouts a week will get a 1.3

- An active job that has three workouts each week will get a 1.4

- An active job that also includes four to five workouts each week will get a 1.5

This is going to give you an idea of what your maintenance calorie intake is. You can just take the number that corresponds with what you do during the week and multiply it with the number that you got above.

After you have this information, it is time to determine your deficit. To do this, you will take the amount that you got before, and then subtract 750 to 250 calories from it. Remember that you will need to burn off 3500 calories in order to lose a pound of body fat. So, depending on how much you take off from the original amount, you can lose between half a pound to one and a half pound. This is a safe range for most people to consistently lose weight, no matter what type of diet plan they are on.

Keep in mind that you can take of more, such as up to 1000 calories each day. But you do need to be careful with this. It can help you to lose weight faster and can be a good idea if you are extremely overweight and need to drop the pounds now. But you do not want to reduce the calories too much, especially while fasting. If you reduce the calories quite a bit, make sure that you are eating lots of healthy and nutrient full ingredients to get the best results and make sure that you keep your body healthy.

This formula should help you to figure out how many calories that you need while on an intermittent fast. It can be changed around for anyone based on their weight, their activity level, and the type of diet they like to enjoy. Make sure to come up with this number before you get started on a fast and then stick with that while you eat on the fast.

Chapter 9:
How to Prepare for Intermittent Fasting

Fasting does not have to be a big deal. While there is a lot of medical advice out there that may tell you that fasting is hard on you, that fasting is impossible to do, and so much more, it is a pretty easy process. Your body is designed to handle fasting, and if you can get past the hunger pains for the first few days, you may find that it isn't as bad as you thought. Plus, you have probably fasted a few times in your life already, and you didn't even realize it. Have you ever had a few days where you were so sick you could barely eat anything? And if you did eat, it was simply a bowl of soup or some crackers? That is basically a short fast by itself.

Now that you know you have already accomplished a few fasts in the past, it is time to learn some simple steps to help you get fully prepared for your fast. Sometimes, learning about fasting and knowing exactly what to expect can be enough to get you ready. Let's look at each one and see how you can prepare for your first intermittent fast.

Learning About Fasting

The first step is to learn more about fasting. You have gone through a lot of this guidebook, so that is a great start. You may also want to consult with your doctor ahead of time too. Fasting can be a great thing for most people, but there can be some medical issues depending on your personal history. And if you are pregnant or nursing, do not start on an intermittent fast. Talking with your doctor is the best way to determine if you are ready to go on a fast so you can really enjoy the benefits, without worrying about your health.

The next step is to determine the type and the length of the fast that you want to practice. There are so many different types of fasting that you can choose, and it often depends on your goals, and which ones you think you can reasonably follow. There are some fasts that include you just drinking water for a few days, some that will be more about juices, some that are all day, or a few days, and some just have you fast every day for a little bit. It is your job to determine which type of fast is the best one for you. Some things to consider about each type of fast include:

Water fasting is one option, but it is a very aggressive form and it is hard to stick with. Most people will not go with this option because it is just too tough to work on. These fasts go from one to forty days, although it is not usually recommended to go the forty days. Usually, ten days is how long someone will choose to go with this type of fast. And it is usually best to start or begin with a juice diet to help.

If you want to go on a liquid diet, it is usually better to go with a juice fast. Juices at least have some calories to them and some other nutrients that can help the body. These juice fasts usually last up to 30 days, but sometimes you will choose to go on this fast for a week or so in order to get yourself started on a new diet plan. You will want to make sure that you are straining out the juices so that you can avoid some of the fibers that will put the digestive system to work and can make you hungrier.

You can also choose to go with something like The Master Cleanse. This is a fast that is kind of a mix between the juice fast and the water fast. You would drink a mixture of maple syrup, water, and fresh lemons and stick with this for about ten minutes. This fast is sometimes easier than the others above because it adds in some calories, but not as many as you might be used to.

A daily fast: This is when you would cut out your foods for so many hours during the day, perhaps going from 16 hours to a few days. You can then eat during some predetermined hours of the day, but for the rest, you only drink some water.

Before you go on the fast, you must make sure that you prepare yourself mentally for some of the changes the body may go through. Fasting is about taking all the toxins out of the body and can help you to lose weight without a lot of hassle. But even with that, it could leave the body feeling weak and a little ill in the beginning. There are also a few other side effects that can show up during the first week or so of the fast, such as headaches, weakness, fatigue, and more. You need to take it slowly and maybe even start your fast while you are off work so you can accommodate your body while it is adjusting.

How to Prepare for a Fast

If you are still trying to decide if you will go on a fast or not, you should do a few other things to prepare. A few weeks before you start on the fast, try to reduce your intake of any addictive or habitual substances that you use. The more that you can reduce these things, the easier the fast is going to be on your whole body. If you smoke or drink alcohol, this is the time to at least reduce your use of them, if not stop them completely. You can also cut down on caffeinated beverages, coffee, soda, and tea as well.

You can also do a test run before you begin the fast. This means you can alter the diet that you already enjoy a few weeks before fasting. This can help your body adjust a little bit, so it isn't in shock when you make the changes. Some tips that you can follow to make this happen includes:

Start eliminating some of the bad stuff a few weeks before. Maybe reduce the baked goods that you enjoy first, and then reduce the soda, and then the processed foods. Go until you are on the diet you wish to follow during the fast.

Start eating smaller portions of meals. This can help the digestive system get used to eating a little less. The meals don't have to be a ton smaller, but a little bit can make a difference and will prepare the stomach.

When you wake up, consider pushing breakfast back a little bit. You don't have to completely cut out your breakfast yet, but maybe push it back an hour or so to help you get used to the change.

If you are going on the Master Fast, then you may want to consider cutting things down a little bit more as you get closer. You can cut down to fruits and vegetables a few days before to help the body get used to the changes. This one can be hard for a lot of people to follow, so unless you have some practice with fasting, it may not be the best option for you to choose.

Knowing What You Should Expect

Sometimes the best thing that you can do for yourself before an intermittent fast is to make sure that you are aware of some of the things that are going to happen during the fast. The first thing to consider is the physical effects the body will go through. The fast is often going to be the most difficult, as well as most uncomfortable, to follow on the first few days. If you have enough willpower to get through those, you will start to feel better and you will be able to get through the fast and see the results.

In the first stage of your fast, which is usually the first two days, you may experience a few side effects until you break the fast and start eating. These side effects can include things like bad breath, a tongue that feels coated, nausea, dizziness, and headaches. These are just the signs that the body is working to cleanse the toxins out of itself. You will probably experience times of being hungry.

In the second stage, which is going to last between days three and seven, your skin may feel a little oily. Some people find that they will break out a little bit. But once you get through that first week, you should be able to see clearer skin.

Sustaining the fast can be a hard thing to do. A lot of time people are going to give up during the first few days because of the discomfort they go through and they feel that it isn't going to get better. Unless you have an actual medical issue that can be worrisome during the fast, breaking the fast early isn't going to benefit the body at all. You aren't going to see the health benefits if you are constantly breaking your fast early and eating a ton of extra food. Some of the things that you can do to help make sure that you don't break out of your fast early includes:

Set the right objective: Before you get started on a fast, take the time to make a clear statement on the reasons you are following a fast. Are you doing it for health reasons, for religious reasons, or just to help you lose weight? You need to set up a clear statement ahead of time so that you can look at it and remember your goals when things get tough.

Make that commitment: Sometimes getting someone, like a friend or a family member, to hold you accountable can make a difference. It can be hard to break out of your fast and quit if someone else is there to monitor you.

Log the fast: As you are getting ready for the fast, you should do some logging and journaling. Write down what you eat during each day, how you are feeling, and what that days' objective is. do this while you are fasting so you can get a good glimpse of how the body is changing.

Chapter 10:
How to Get Back on Track if You Fall Off the Fast

There are times when staying with an intermittent fast, or any other type of diet plan when things can get hard. You may have a cheat day here or there. That is perfectly normal, and sometimes it can even be a healthy and effective way to stay on your diet plan. But then there are other times when you will completely fall off the intermittent fast, and you may not follow it for weeks, or months, or even more.

When you fall off the intermittent fast, you may be curious about how you should get back on track. You want to get the best results possible, but there is some worry that you will fail again. And no one wants to jump into the fasting again with the thought that they might fail.

No matter what kind of diet plan you go on, there may come a time when you fall off your plan. You may have done well for some time, but then you got lazy, decided to take a break, had a stressful situation occur, or something else that caused you to drop the intermittent fast and not follow it anymore. But the trick to seeing weight loss and better health over the long term is to just get back on plan any time that you start falling off. Luckily, there are a few different things that you can do to help you get back on track when you fall off your intermittent fast:

Analyze Your Plan

The first thing that you do is analyze the plan that you are going to follow. Which intermittent fast do you plan to be on? Did you have a meal plan to work with? Some of the steps you can do here include:

- Did you have a plan that was written out? If you didn't, then now is the time to get it out on paper.

- Ask yourself if this plan was just too hard for you. If you had tried to do the Warrior diet, maybe going with a different option is better. Maybe doing the Leangains plan every other day would be better. You can switch from a 24-hour fast to a 16/8 plan. Mix it up to work better for you.

- If you think that the plan you picked was too easy and you aren't getting the results that you want, then it is time to move to the second step.

Perform a Postmortem

- Ask yourself why you ended up falling off the plan. Be serious with yourself. Then you can take the right actions in order to solve these problems.

- If you found that the major problem you had with intermittent fasting is eating during the fasting time, then ask yourself the following questions

- Was I hungry when I ate? If you are dealing with true hunger and that is why you broke the fast, and this happens often, then it may be time to increase the amount that you eat during your feeding window, or lengthen that time frame a bit more.

- Was I bored? Boredom can be a big reason why we feel hungry during our fasts. Find some interests or get a hobby, or just get out of the house and see if that helps.

- Was I stressed out? If you are stressed, find some way to relieve that stress. Talk to somebody, go out for a nice walk, or spend time journaling.

- Was I tired? If this is your problem, make sure that you get more sleep. You can consider taking a nap the next time you are hungry rather than eating.

Find Motivation to Help You Get Back on the Plan

Now you need to figure out why you went off your intermittent fasting plan. Sometimes just figuring this out is going to help you be motivated and can help you get to the right solution. But if you need some other type of motivation, then you need to find that for you.

To come up with the motivation, figure out why you want to go on an intermittent fast. Was it to lose weight? Was it to get more energy? Did you want to improve some health condition and thought intermittent fasting would be the right way to do this? Then think about what would happen if you didn't reach that goal? This can often be enough to motivate you to get back on track. There are many different types of motivations that you can rely on including:

- Wanting to lose weight to look and feel better.

- To improve your risk of type 2 diabetes.

- To have more energy to keep up with the kids

- To improve your lifespan

- To prevent aging

- To reduce your risk of developing cancer later in life.

- To make your brain sharper

And if you find that your previous motivation wasn't enough to keep you going, then it may be time to think of a new motivation to try out. This can be anything that you want, if it helps you to stay on the fast and do well.

Ultimately, you need to realize that when you fall off your plan of intermittent fasting, and you are considering getting back on it, you are technically at a crossroads. You can choose to quit right now, or you can go back to where you were. You can also choose to be stubborn and then press on some more. The choice is yours, but you need to be the one to make that decision and stick with it once you do.

Chapter 11:
Exercising While Intermittent Fasting

The next topic we are going to look at is exercising while you are on an intermittent fast. Many people go on one of these fasts in the hopes of losing weight. And while the diet you follow is going to do wonders for weight loss, you often need to add in some form of exercise to help tone up and really see the results. But if you are new to intermittent fasting, you may be worried about how this type of eating is going to affect your workouts, and if it is even safe to do a workout on the fast. Let's look at some of the specifics of working out on an intermittent fast and how to do this safely.

When Should I Exercise?

The next question is when you should exercise. Many people are confused about the best time for exercising when they are on an intermittent fast. They may choose to exercise during their eating window because they assume the body will need that fuel or that they will be too tired to exercise during the fast. But, the best time to exercise is during that fast.

When you exercise during the fast, your body has already spent some time burning through the readily available glucose in the body and has started working on the glycogen and excess fat. When you add in exercise currently, you are forcing the body to burn through more stored fat to provide you with the energy that you need. This results in faster and better weight loss results than exercising at any other time.

After the workout is done, it is a good idea to break your fast. This allows you to get in some nutrients that help the body repair itself after the workout. Make sure that it is well-balanced with some healthy fats and some protein (along with some carbs, even if you are on the ketogenic diet). This helps the body repair itself after the workout and can replace some of the nutrients that you lost during the workout.

Exercising During Your Fast Speeds Up Weight Loss.
If you are trying to lose weight, then exercising all on its own is not going to be the answer. There are many people who will go all out on the exercise portion of weight loss, but then they won't spend any time trying to fix their eating habits. There are countless studies that state how exercise has very little effect on your personal body weight, at least on its own.

However, when you combine exercise with an intermittent fast, it can help to boost the amount of weight loss that you see. This is because, when you are in your fast, the body has run out of readily available glucose, and it has turned to the stored fat in the body for fuel. If you decide to exercise while the body is in this state, you will burn through more fat compared to exercising during your eating window.

In addition, exercising during your fast can also help improve the way that the body is able to handle the carbs that are there. This can lead to a reduction in your risk for diabetes. All in all, exercising during a fast can help you lose weight while also improving your overall health.

Exercising During a Fast Will Improve Your Performance.

Working out before you have breakfast, or before you end your fast, has been found in several studies to improve your performance. The changes that will take place in your metabolism and with your muscles are amazing, and they are going to improve your fitness and will happen more quickly while also improving your muscle growth.

Can Improve Your Muscle Repair and Stops the Hunger Pains

One study that was done on mice found that when they exercised while in a fasted stated, it helped them to improve their repair process of the muscles. This is especially true when the repair is compared to exercising in the fed state, or during your eating windows.

In addition, many experienced fasters know that when they exercise on one of their fasting days, it is a good way to stop some of the hunger pains they are feeling. There is also some scientific research that confirms how exercising when you are hungry can make the hunger pains go away.

What Exercises are the Best?

The good news is that the benefits you get with adding exercise to your fast will count whether you are doing weight training, HIIT, or lower intensity workouts. The experts would say that you should try to do some mixture of all three to get the best benefits to your health. However, the best type of exercise is the kind that you enjoy because you are more likely to stick with that exercise, rather than stopping. Pick out the type of exercise that you like the most, and then use that during your fast.

One thing to note is that some types of exercise are sometimes harder to do during a long fast, meaning they are going to be difficult for you to do during the end of a fasting day. For example, HIIT exercises can be great options to improve your health, but they do need some carbs stored in the body to accomplish. The body won't be able to burn fat fast enough to do these exercises, so they are sometimes hard to do, especially over longer periods of time, compared to the other workouts. If you want to do HIIT, consider doing it early in the fast to avoid these issues.

Weightlifting is usually pretty easy to do during the fasting time. You will want to do this one near the end of the fasting time so you can break the fast and eat afterwards. You need to get in some healthy nutrients shortly after your weightlifting session to ensure that the muscles get the nutrition, they need to not get damaged.

If you want an exercise that you can do no matter what time of your fast it is, then go with something that is low intensity. This could include various exercises, such as walking. Walking, at least low intensity walking isn't going to use up your stored glycogen and can be done any time that you would like.

HIIT

If you don't feel like spending all that time and all those hours outside running or in the gym, or you want to make sure that you are maximizing the health benefits that you get from exercise, then adding in some high intensity interval training to your routine can be just what you need.

Research has found that doing three rounds of high intensity exercise, with each round being between 20 seconds to a minute, done three times a week, can have as many beneficial effects on your body as running on the treadmill for an hour. This means you could just take a few minutes each day and get the same benefits, without all the time and energy of the gym.

Give Your Body Sometime to Adapt

Exercise is great for you. Even if you are not trying to lose a lot of weight, exercise can be good for the mind, body, and weight loss. And while fasting and exercise can be the best of friends, it is not a good idea to go hardcore when you first get started.

For most people, the first few days, and even up to the first week, can be hard on a fast. You are trying to get your body adapted to a new way of eating, and this can take some time. Add in the hunger pains, the cravings, and just getting used to a new schedule, and it is all hard to do.

For the first few fasts, do not exercise heavily. Until you have had a chance to try out a fast, you won't know how the body is going to react. If you find that you can adapt quickly and fasting doesn't seem to be a big deal, then it is fine to add in the exercise program and see how it goes.

Walking

Walking is always a good workout to help you lose weight, but it is especially good when you are on an intermittent fast. It helps you to burn calories, get moving, and can get you outside so you aren't so distracted by all the food around you during a fasting time.

The amount of time that you stand up and walk around, compared to the amount of time that you sit, can have a big impact on your health and your weight loss. The amount of time that you stand up and move around, known as the NEAT non-exercise activity thermogenesis). It is agreed that overall,

NEAT is going to contribute more to how much energy is used than formal exercises. This means that if you can increase the NEAT level you have, it is easier to lose weight faster. This should be an easy thing to see. Who usually seems to be in better health; someone who spends all their day sitting or one who is up and, on their feet, even if they don't' do formal exercise?

If you are having trouble motivating yourself to do a workout, then remember that NEAT could still be the option for you. Increase your NEAT score on both the fasting and the feasting days. Set an alarm that alerts you every hour and get up and walk around for a few minutes. Go outside and take a walk around the block a few times. The intensity doesn't have to be that high, just if you are up and moving a little bit, rather than sitting around.

Chapter 12:
Tips to Stay Motivated and Success

The good news is that working with an intermittent fast is a simple process to use. Considering all the great benefits you can get from this kind of eating plan; you are going to find that it is easier than some of the other diet plans you may have tried. And there are so many options of intermittent fasts that you can choose, that you are sure to find the option that works the best for your lifestyle or your preferences.

If you are new to the idea of intermittent fast, then it is important to know exactly how you should get started. Here are a few tips that you can use to help you get the most out of your intermittent fast.

Be Careful About the Kind of Exercise You Do

In the beginning, when you are getting used to a fast, you need to be careful about the types of exercises that you choose to do. You are going to be tired and getting adjusted to this new way of eating. Doing some intense workouts can really take a toll on the body. As a beginner, it may be best if you simply try out the fasting and see how your body reacts, and then add in the working out later.

If you do plan to do some intense workouts while fasting, then you do need to take your time. You may find that you need to adjust your fasting window, change up the diet you are on, or make sure that you are doing the workouts at the right time to make them work.

Learn How to Listen to Your Body
One thing that you will learn to do with this kind of fast is how to listen to your body. Through the years, many of us have learned how to eat just because it is time to eat. When lunch time rolls around, we eat, regardless of if we're hungry or not. The same happens with breakfast, dinner, and even the snacks. We eat because we have been told for our whole lives that this is the time to eat, and we don't really pay attention to if we are hungry during that time. We just choose to eat.

This is a bad habit to get into. We eat because we think we need to, rather than listening to our bodies and eating when we are hungry. This leads to a lot of grazing during the day, overeating, and can make us out of tun with our bodies. Intermittent fasting works to fix this issue.

When you are on this fast, you are going to learn to listen to your body. You will go through fasting periods, so you better learn when your body is hungry. Then, when you break the fast, you will eat until you feel satisfied. If you have a day where you need a little less food, then you eat less. You don't eat just because it is time.

Doing this has several benefits. You will learn how to listen to your body. You will eat when your body wants you to, not because the clock says it is time. This helps you to reduce the calories that you consume and can be much healthier. It also helps you to listen to your body, and you may be able to tell when there are other issues happening as well.

Meal Planning Can Make It Easier
Sometimes the best thing to do during a fast is to bring out your favorite recipes and create a meal plan. Meal planning can take some of the work out of the week, which can be especially important on a fast. When you are done with a fast, you will feel hungry, and it's not likely you will make the best nutritional decisions when the fast ends. With a meal plan, you can have the meals prepared and ready to go. You know exactly what you are going to eat, and when, to save the hassle and to ensure you stick to the fast, and the right calorie amounts, even when you feel hungry.

Meal planning can take any form that you want. Some choose to follow something like the ketogenic diet to lose more weight and will make sure they have lots of meals and snacks on hand to help them stick with that when they are hungry. Others will do the same, but with a different diet plan like the Paleo, Mediterranean, or DASH diets.

You don't have to stick with a specific diet though. You can choose to just eat healthy foods and meals, and then create a meal plan that meets up with this. Simply having healthy foods on hand can make it easier to stay on an intermittent fast.

Drink Plenty of Fluids
One thing that you need to remember when going on an intermittent fast is to drink plenty of fluids. But when you are in your fasting period, you need to

make sure that you get enough fluids to prevent dehydration and to help your body function properly.

Many times, when we are not eating, we fail to get in enough fluids to keep us going. Our body will often respond with more hunger pains in the hopes of getting you to drink something. But then we will assume that we are just feeling hungry and will want to eat even more than before. When you are on the fast, feeling hungry from not eating and from lack of hydration can be hard during this time.

Any time that you feel hungry on an intermittent fast, make sure to drink some liquids. It is likely that this is enough to help you feel better without having to break your fast and eat anything. Water is often the best option to go with here, but you can also pick coffee and other beverages that don't have calories in them to help mix things up a little bit.

Get Out of the House with Some Fun Distractions
If you are sitting around the house, thinking about food, it is going to be a million times harder to stick with your intermittent fast. There is probably plenty of food around the house, and the more you think about that food, the harder it is to resist the food. And the longer you sit around the house, the harder it will be to resist the temptation to eat, and the more miserable you will be if you don't eat at that time.

The best thing to do is find a way to keep yourself distracted. Get out of the house and go do something. You can choose to go on a walk. Head to the library and spend some time reading some of your favorite books. Go and spend some time with friends. If it keeps you busy and gets you out of the house, it is going to help.

Find Ways to Reduce Your Stress

It can be hard to do a fast when you are feeling a lot of stress. You will have some extra cravings, and if you are dealing with all the stresses in your life, it can be extra difficult to deal with these cravings. While an intermittent fast is not meant to be difficult, it can sometimes be hard to stick with it when you are also dealing with stress.

Since you can't completely get rid of all the stress that you feel in your life, it is better if you learn some effective methods to help you relieve stress when it comes up. You can set up a good exercise routine that helps you to naturally release stress when you feel it coming on. Many people like to practice mindfulness or meditation to get rid of stress. Options like going on a walk, spending time with friends, taking a warm bath, reading a book, and more can help you to reduce your stress so that you can stay on your intermittent fast without worry.

Find a Friend Who Will Do the Fast with You

Sometimes, the best way to get the most out of your intermittent fast is to find someone who is willing to go on the fast with you. Going on an intermittent fast on your own can be tough. You may feel that no one else understands what you are going through, and there is going to be a lot of temptation out there against you.

But if you have someone to work on the fast with you, it can be easier. Both of you can be there to support each other. When you run into a time that is particularly tough, that friend can be a good support person to stand behind you and help you stay on track. Everything is better when you do it with a friend so consider asking someone to be there along with you.

Don't Have a Big Last Supper
Another thing that you should be careful about is not gorging yourself with a final big feast before you fast. The night before, pick out a meal that is healthy and can help keep you full throughout some of your fast. This means, pick out a mean that has a lot of great vegetables, lots of healthy fat, and some lean protein.

Starches, such as legumes or a sweet potato, can be nice for your meal as well. And don't forget to add in some fruits to your meals to provide it with some natural sugar, something that is very calming to your hormones. Berries are often the best here because they are low on the glycemic index.

Make the Fast Fit into Your Current Lifestyle
Before you get started on a fast, think about it a little bit. You don't want to fast during times when you are going to deal with a lot of stress. You also don't want to fast during events that will cause a lot of extra exertion on your part. These are times that are hard to fast because the cravings can be tough, and you may need more energy to get through them.

You can also plan your fasting around the times that work for you. For example, if you are on the 5:2 diet or another 24-hour diet, pick days when you are going to be busy anyway. You will be too busy to really notice that you haven't eaten much. And you can even take some of the stress out of your day by not having to worry about food and making a meal on top of everything else.

Make Sure That You Are Fit Enough to Fast
While intermittent fasting can be a good thing for a lot of different people, there are some people who shouldn't fast. Those who shouldn't be fasting

include any child under 18 years old, anyone who has some serious medical conditions, and pregnant or breastfeeding women.

In addition, if you are taking some prescription medications, you should talk to your doctor before you get started with an intermittent fast. Sometimes these medications can cause some bad side effects when you are on a fast. If you are not able to get on a fast, you should consider going on a cleaner eating diet to get some weight loss results as well.

There are a lot of different ways to do an intermittent fast, which is part of why it is so liked by many different people. If you are considering an intermittent fast, take the time to look through this chapter and see what some of the best tips and tricks are for you to try out for the best results.

Chapter 13:
Common Questions

1. Which type of intermittent fasting should I choose and why?

There are many intermittent fasting regiments but the most common is the 16:8 where you fast for 16 hours and have an eating window of 8 hours. Typically, this plan works well for most individuals and the least challenging to fit within your daily lives. However, if you're up for the challenge, the warrior diet, alternate day fasting or even a weekly 24-hour fast is suitable. If you're getting the calories and nutrients that are required of your body, then no harm will be done.

2. How and what should I eat during feeding periods?

The beauty of intermittent fasting is you are not told what to eat but when to eat. The rule of thumb is to get the nutrients and protein needed daily first. Afterward, your goal is to fulfill the daily calorie intake to weight lose weight or maintain your weight.

3. I'm really concerned about losing muscle mass. How can I prevent this from happening while training and fasting intermittently?

In order not to lose muscle mass you must intake enough protein, so muscle is not broken down due to a deficient in protein. Some find it best to eat after working out but again, if your intake your protein requirement than muscle breakdown will not occur.

4. I'm not fasting to lose WEIGHT; how do I manage to eat enough food during my feeding window?

This is entirely based on the nutrients needed to maintain your weight. If your daily calorie intake is about 1800 calories, then you must fit that into your eating window. The foods you eat are entirely up to you. You can decide what foods to eat, but they must take up your daily maintenance calorie intake to not lose weight.

5. Fasting for all those hours seem overwhelming, what can I do to make it easier?

There are many methods described in the book, but the most common is to have busy work. Keep your mind from drifting and thinking about food. Find hobbies or change your environment, so you are not surrounded by food.

6. How do I coordinate my training schedule for my intermittent fasting schedule?

The most common is to train before breaking your fast. Most people find this to be the most rewarding because after an intense workout you can reward yourself with the foods you want to eat.

7. Is it ok to drink diet soda when I fast intermittently?

You may drink diet soda if and only if it contains zero calories. However, there are conflicting studies that report too much artificial sweeteners may trigger insulin negating the benefits of fasting. For now, you may drink diet soda but keep it to a minimum of no more than two.

8. Can I and should I take vitamins while intermittent fasting?
There is no harm in taking multivitamins during any intermittent fasting regiment. The goal during your eating window is to consume the necessary nutrients, protein, carbs, and calories to achieve your desired results.

9. Why would anyone fast who doesn't want to lose weight?
Fasting is not only used for weight loss. The many benefits of fasting include reduced insulin resistance, improve your heart health, improve brain function, increase HGH production, and let us not forget that it allows us to have a simple eating schedule. These are only a few but as we continue to research the benefits of fasting, more and more benefits will be revealed.

10. How should I prepare myself to fast intermittently?
Typically, how most individuals begin is to decrease there eating window every few days. This allows your body to adjust. Jumping right into a 16:8 fast can be challenging but incrementally working your way towards the schedule is how most individuals maintain fasting long term.

11. Why do I get headaches when I fast and how can I stop them?
There is not a straightforward answer for this. Research has shown some triggers can be due to low blood sugar or other medical conditions. If fasting triggers headaches, then consult a medical professional to isolate the cause.

12. Isn't intermittent fasting a fancy way of saying I'm starving myself?

Intermittent fast is not a form of starvation. During your eating window, your goal is to consume the necessary foods to meet your daily nutrients, proteins, and calories. When you starve yourself, you are not getting the nutrients you need.

13. I've heard intermittent fasting isn't safe for women, what are the facts?

Intermittent fasting is perfectly safe for women. Certain medical conditions require you to eat frequently but outside of these medical conditions there should not be an issue. For peace in mind, you should consult a medical professional about any medical conditions you feel would have adverse effects while intermittent fasting.

14. Why can't I have a protein shake when I'm fasting?

Protein shakes have calories that require breakdown during digestion. This triggers an insulin reaction which is the opposite desired effect during your fast.

15. How can I fast while I'm on vacation?

This is quite simple, only eat during your eating window. Maintain self-discipline and do not gorge on everything you come across. Although you're on vacation, this doesn't mean you can break the fasting rules.

16. Can intermittent fasting really be a long-term weight loss solution?

Of course, it can. In fact, our ancestors fasted instead of eating throughout the day. They would consume an enormous daily meal. Intermittent fasting is not harmful; therefore, it can be a long-term weight loss solution.

17. Can I stop fasting once I reach my weight goal?

Personally, if fasting is a nuisance, then this is not the weight regiment for you. There are many other options to assist with weight loss. Intermittent fasting is a popular choice, but it all comes down to personal preference. If you're able to maintain your weight loss without fasting, then there is no reason why you can't stop intermittent fasting. If it's bothersome for you, then pick another weight loss plan.

Conclusion

The next step is to get started on your own intermittent fast. As we explained in this guidebook, there are a lot of different versions of an intermittent fast that you can choose to go on, which makes it perfect for anyone who is trying to lose weight. Whether you want to go a whole day without eating, or you find that a small fast on most days of the week is best for you, you can really see some amazing results with intermittent fasting.

This guidebook took some time to go through the basics of intermittent fasting and to help prepare you for using this kind of eating plan in your own life. Whether you are looking to lose weight, decrease your risk of developing diabetes, help you to improve your heart health, or something else, this is the best eating plan for you. It gives you a lot of choices, a lot of freedom, and you will still see results.

If you find this book helpful in anyway a review to support my endeavors is much appreciated.

Christine Moore

www.ingramcontent.com/pod-product-compliance
Lightning Source LLC
Chambersburg PA
CBHW020301030426
42336CB00010B/853